ALLERGY ALLEVIATION

Advanced Therapies For Respiratory And Skin Allergies

Find Relief From Allergies Through Cutting-Edge Therapies Targeting Both Respiratory And Skin-Related Allergic Reactions

DR. BRIDGET PROMISE

Table of Contents

CHAPTER ONE

Introduction

Allergies are a common and sometimes misunderstood health issue that affects millions of individuals worldwide. The immune system, which protects the body from dangerous chemicals, may sometimes misidentify innocuous materials as dangers.

This misidentification activates the body's defensive systems, resulting in what we typically refer to as an allergic response.

Understanding Allergies

To understand allergies, we must first understand how the immune system works. The immune system's principal function is to identify and eliminate possible dangers including bacteria, viruses, and poisons. However, in those with allergies, this defensive system fails. Instead of protecting the body from true dangers, the immune system responds to largely innocuous substances as invaders.

Allergic responses occur when the immune system creates antibodies, particularly immunoglobulin E (IgE), in response to an allergen. These antibodies, in turn, produce different substances, including histamines, which cause the symptoms often linked with allergies.

Basics Of Respiratory And Skin Allergies

Allergies may take many forms, with respiratory and skin allergies being among the most common. Respiratory allergies affect both the upper and lower respiratory tracts, generating symptoms such as sneezing, nasal congestion, coughing, and wheezing. Pollen, dust mites, pet dander, and mold spores are among the most common respiratory allergens.

Skin allergies, on the other hand, are caused by allergens coming into contact with the skin, resulting in symptoms like itching, redness, and rashes. Common skin allergies include some metals, latex, particular materials, and other compounds found in skincare or housekeeping goods.

Identify Triggers: Common Allergens

Recognizing and identifying allergens is critical for successful allergy treatment. Common allergies are divided into three categories: airborne allergens, food allergens, and contact allergens.

Airborne allergens include tree, grass, and weed pollen, mold spores, and pet dander. Understanding the seasonal changes and common allergies in your area might help you minimize exposure.

Nuts, seafood, dairy products, and some fruits are among the most prevalent food allergies. Identifying and removing particular items from your diet may greatly reduce allergy responses.

touch allergens are compounds that induce skin allergies when in direct touch. These may include metals such as nickel, which is prevalent in jewelry, as well as compounds found in cosmetics, soaps, and detergents.

Traditional Allergy Management

Allergies are managed using a mix of preventative techniques and treatment alternatives. Traditional allergy management methods include over-the-counter medicines and prescription therapies.

Over-the-counter medications

Over-the-counter (OTC) drugs are widely accessible without a prescription and may alleviate mild to severe allergy symptoms. Antihistamines, such as cetirizine (Zyrtec) and loratadine (Claritin), function by inhibiting histamine activity, decreasing symptoms such as sneezing, itching, and runny nose.

Decongestants, such as pseudoephedrine, reduce nasal congestion by restricting blood vessels. However, they should be taken with caution since long-term usage might cause rebound congestion.

Nasal sprays with corticosteroids, such as fluticasone (Flonase) or budesonide (Rhinocort), may successfully decrease inflammation in the nasal passages, relieving congestion and other nasal symptoms.

CHAPTER TWO

Prescription Treatments For Allergies

Individuals with severe or chronic allergies may need prescription drugs. Prescription antihistamines, decongestants, and nasal corticosteroids are often more strong than over-the-counter alternatives and may be prescribed when OTC treatments are inadequate.

In situations of persistent or severe allergic responses, allergists may recommend immunotherapy. This therapy consists of progressively exposing the person to increasing doses of the allergen to desensitize the immune system over time. Immunotherapy may be given as allergy injections or sublingual pills.

In emergency instances requiring quick treatment, healthcare practitioners may prescribe epinephrine auto-injectors. These devices provide a quick dose of epinephrine, a hormone that treats severe allergic responses including anaphylaxis.

Allergies are a complicated and prevalent health condition that has a substantial influence on individuals who suffer from them.

Understanding the fundamentals of allergies, such as their causes and typical triggers, is critical for successful treatment. Respiratory and skin allergies are the most common types of allergic responses, each with its own set of symptoms.

Identifying common allergens, whether airborne, food-related, or contact-based, is critical for avoiding triggers and reducing allergy responses. Traditional allergy care techniques include both preventative and treatment measures. Over-the-counter drugs may relieve moderate symptoms, but prescription treatments may be required for more severe instances.

Finally, consulting with healthcare specialists, especially allergists, may assist patients in developing tailored allergy treatment programs. Whether via medication, immunotherapy, or lifestyle changes, good allergy management allows people to live healthier, more comfortable lives despite their allergic sensitivity.

Respiratory allergies may have a substantial influence on people's quality of life, limiting their ability to breathe freely and participate in regular activities without pain. As medical research advances, so do the therapy options for respiratory allergies. This article looks at advanced therapeutics, with a special emphasis on immunotherapy for respiratory allergies and new medicines. It also covers sophisticated treatments for skin allergies, such as topical treatments and phototherapy.

Immunotherapy: Allergy Shots.

Immunotherapy, often known as allergy injections, is a proven and successful treatment for respiratory allergies. To desensitize the immune system, allergens are administered in steadily increasing amounts. The idea is to teach the immune system to accept certain allergens that cause allergic responses.

Allergy injections are usually indicated for those who have moderate to severe allergies and have not found relief from other therapies. The method starts with an allergy test to determine which allergens impact the person. Once identified, a tailored vaccination is manufactured using modest doses of these allergens.

Patients are given vaccination shots regularly, starting with higher doses and then decreasing them over time. This mechanism permits the immune system to adapt and become tolerant to allergens. Individuals often find a reduction in allergy symptoms as well as a decrease in the requirement for additional allergy treatments.

Immunotherapy is very effective for respiratory allergies such as hay fever, allergic rhinitis, and asthma. It treats the underlying source of allergies by modulating the immunological response, offering long-term relief to many people.

Sublingual Immunotherapy (Slit).

Sublingual immunotherapy (SLIT) is an alternative to standard allergy injections. Instead of injections, SLIT involves putting a little number of allergen extracts beneath your tongue. This procedure is more convenient for people who are afraid of needles or have trouble attending normal clinic appointments.

Similar to allergy injections, SLIT works by exposing the immune system to modest, regulated doses of allergen. Over time, this exposure helps the body develop tolerance, lowering the intensity of allergic responses. SLIT is often used to treat respiratory allergies such as pollen, dust mites, and pet dander.

One of the benefits of SLIT is its administrative flexibility. Patients may use the sublingual allergen extract at home, which reduces the need for frequent clinic visits. Individuals seeking SLIT should talk with their healthcare physician to establish if it is a viable choice depending on their unique sensitivities and medical history.

Emerging Treatments And Research

As medical science develops, new and creative treatment options for respiratory allergies arise. Researchers are looking at several techniques to alter the immune response and give tailored relief to allergy sufferers.

One interesting field of study is biologics, which are genetically modified proteins generated from human DNA. These biologics target particular immune system components that cause allergic responses. By targeting the underlying processes of allergies, biologics have the potential to provide more effective and focused therapy with fewer adverse effects.

Furthermore, continuing study looks at the use of nanoparticles to deliver allergens in a controlled way. This technique intends to improve immunotherapy accuracy and efficiency, possibly lowering treatment time and increasing overall results for patients with respiratory allergies.

Advanced Treatments For Skin Allergies

In addition to respiratory allergies, skin allergies are a major health problem for many people. Advanced skin allergy treatments address the underlying causes while also delivering tailored symptom alleviation.

CHAPTER THREE

Topical Solutions For Allergic Skin Conditions

Topical therapies are essential for controlling allergic skin diseases such as eczema, contact dermatitis, and hives. Corticosteroid creams and ointments are routinely used to treat inflammation and irritation. However, long-term usage of corticosteroids may cause negative effects, prompting the investigation of alternate therapies.

Calcineurin inhibitors, which affect the immunological response in the skin, are among the most advanced topical therapies. These lotions and ointments help manage inflammation while avoiding the adverse effects associated with long-term corticosteroid usage. They are especially effective in managing chronic skin diseases and preventing flare-ups.

Phototherapy: Light-Based Approaches

Phototherapy, often known as light therapy, is a sophisticated treatment for specific types of skin allergies. It entails exposing the damaged skin to certain wavelengths of light, either from natural sunshine or artificial light sources. This method is very beneficial for illnesses including psoriasis, eczema, and vitiligo.

UV light is often utilized in phototherapy, and treatments may be provided in a medical environment or at home. Controlled UV light exposure regulates immunological responses in the skin, lowering inflammation and encouraging healing.

While phototherapy may be very efficient, it must be closely monitored to avoid unwanted adverse effects such as sunburn and an increased risk of skin cancer. Individuals getting phototherapy must follow their healthcare provider's advice and attend frequent check-ups.

In conclusion, innovative medicines for respiratory and skin allergies have considerably enhanced the treatment options for those suffering from these disorders. Immunotherapy, whether administered by allergy injections or sublingual techniques, is a critical component in treating the underlying causes of respiratory allergies. Ongoing research and developing medicines, including biologics and nanoparticle-based therapeutics, offer the potential for more tailored and effective therapy.

Advanced topical therapies for skin allergies, such as calcineurin inhibitors, give alternatives to standard corticosteroids, while phototherapy uses light to modulate the immune system. As medical research advances, people suffering from respiratory and skin allergies should expect increasingly effective and individualized treatment choices, improving their overall well-being and quality of life.

In recent years, the area of dermatological allergy treatment has undergone a paradigm change, with new techniques developing to successfully treat allergic diseases. Beyond standard treatments, a complete strategy also includes lifestyle changes to alleviate allergies. This comprehensive approach includes allergen avoidance tactics, nutritional recommendations, and the development of allergy-friendly living settings.

Allergen Avoidance Strategies

Allergen avoidance methods are a key component of modern dermatological allergy therapy.

Identifying and reducing allergen exposure is critical for successful allergy management. This method goes beyond topical treatments to include lifestyle changes that may have a substantial influence on an individual's overall well-being.

Understanding the individual allergens that cause dermatological responses is critical. Dermatologists may use extensive allergy testing to correctly identify these triggers. Once diagnosed, patients may take proactive steps to avoid contact with these allergies. Individuals who are sensitive to specific metals present in jewelry, for example, may choose hypoallergenic or nickel-free options.

Furthermore, lifestyle changes influence clothing choices. Wool and synthetic fabrics may worsen dermatological allergies. Choosing breathable, natural fibers such as cotton may assist in alleviating skin irritation and pain. Furthermore, wearing protective clothes, such as long sleeves and helmets, might function as a barrier to environmental allergens.

Dietary Concerns For Allergy Relief

The link between nutrition and dermatological allergens is gaining popularity in modern medical discourse. Certain foods may aggravate allergic skin issues, whilst others might improve general skin health. Dermatologists are increasingly emphasizing the importance of dietary choices in allergy alleviation.

Nuts, dairy, shellfish, and gluten are among the most common allergens. Individuals with dermatological allergies should undergo food sensitivity testing to identify specific triggers. Once diagnosed, a specific dietary plan may be developed to prevent or restrict the intake of these allergies.

In contrast, consuming foods with anti-inflammatory characteristics may aid with allergy relief. Omega-3 fatty acids, which are present in fatty fish such as salmon, as well as antioxidants from fruits and vegetables, help to maintain skin health and may reduce allergic responses. A well-balanced and nutrient-dense diet is essential for maintaining good skin and boosting the body's natural allergy defense mechanisms.

Developing An Allergy-Friendly Home Environment

Individuals may exercise great control over their exposure to allergens in their own homes. Creating an allergy-friendly home environment needs serious consideration in many parts of everyday life.

Regular cleaning is essential since dust mites, pet dander, and mold are major indoor allergies. Hypoallergenic bedding, frequent cleaning of carpets and upholstery, and sufficient ventilation may all help to create a cleaner interior environment. In addition, using air purifiers with HEPA filters may successfully minimize airborne allergens.

Another important component of maintaining an allergy-friendly home is carefully selecting cosmetics and housekeeping items. Choosing fragrance-free and hypoallergenic products reduces the chance of skin discomfort. Checking ingredient labels for allergies and avoiding harsh chemicals may help improve skin health.

Holistic Approaches To Allergy Elimination

Holistic methods for allergy relief emphasize the interdependence of several parts of a person's life. These techniques aim to improve total well-being rather than only treating particular symptoms, acknowledging that stress, sleep, and mental health may all have an impact on allergic disorders.

Stress management strategies, such as mindfulness meditation and yoga, have shown the potential to lower the intensity of allergic skin responses. Stress may aggravate inflammatory reactions, making people more prone to allergy flare-ups. Incorporating relaxation activities into everyday routines may help to improve overall skin health.

Adequate sleep is another important aspect of holistic allergy treatment. Poor sleep quality may weaken the immune system, making people more prone to allergic responses. Establishing a regular sleep schedule and establishing a pleasant sleeping environment may improve both sleep quality and overall dermatological health.

Furthermore, mental health factors influence allergy treatment. Emotions may affect conditions like eczema and psoriasis. Integrating mental health assistance, such as counseling or therapy, into allergy treatment may help with the psychological elements of dermatological diseases while also improving general well-being.

Finally, emerging techniques in dermatological allergy care stress a holistic viewpoint that goes beyond standard therapies. Lifestyle changes, such as allergen avoidance techniques, dietary considerations, and developing allergy-friendly living settings, are critical components of modern allergy treatment. Individuals who take a holistic approach may actively engage in treating their dermatological allergies and enhancing their overall quality of life.

Mind-Body Techniques: Meditation And Stress Management

In today's fast-paced, often stressful environment, controlling allergies entails more than just treating physical symptoms. Mind-body strategies in allergy treatment have received a lot of attention since they take a holistic approach to total health. Meditation and stress management are two important components of this strategy since they help to reduce the effect of allergies on both the body and the mind.

Individuals dealing with allergies might benefit greatly from meditation. Allergies may cause a variety of physical and mental symptoms, ranging from nasal congestion to increased anxiety. Individuals may build a higher level of awareness and mindfulness by engaging in regular meditation activities. As a result, they are better able to detect and react to allergens.

Mindfulness meditation, a technique with ancient roots, is paying complete attention to the present moment without passing judgment. For allergy patients, this entails noticing symptoms without letting them dominate one's thinking. This allows people to interrupt the cycle of concern and anxiety that is often connected with allergies, encouraging a feeling of serenity and control.

In addition to mindfulness meditation, different relaxation methods may be used to reduce stress, which is a typical trigger for allergies. Progressive muscle relaxation, deep breathing techniques, and guided visualization are all strategies for promoting relaxation and relieving stress. Individuals who incorporate these activities into their everyday routines will lower overall stress levels, which will improve their allergy symptoms.

CHAPTER FIVE

Alternative Treatments In Allergy Management

Beyond traditional treatments, alternative medicines have emerged as effective allergy control solutions. These techniques understand the body's interconnection and aim to treat the underlying reasons for allergic responses.

While alternative treatments are not a substitute for medical guidance, they may supplement traditional therapy and bring relief to those looking for new methods of allergy management.

Acupuncture, an ancient Chinese method of inserting small needles into particular places on the body, has shown potential in treating allergy problems.

Acupuncture proponents think that it helps to realign the body's energy flow, increasing general health and minimizing allergic responses. According to scientific research, acupuncture may have anti-inflammatory properties, making it a potentially useful supplement to allergy care measures.

Herbal medicine is another alternative treatment gaining

popularity in the field of allergy control. Certain plants, such as butterbur and stinging nettle, offer anti-allergic effects. Butterbur, in particular, has been examined for its ability to alleviate symptoms of allergic rhinitis. Before introducing herbal medicines into allergy therapy, consumers should check with a healthcare practitioner to establish their safety and effectiveness.

Integrating Holistic Practices With Conventional Care

Holistic approaches include treating the whole person—mind, body, and spirit—rather than just particular symptoms. Integrating holistic techniques into standard allergy therapy may improve overall health and treatment efficacy. Holistic treatment stresses the role of lifestyle variables such as nutrition, exercise, and stress management in controlling allergic diseases.

Dietary changes, such as following an anti-inflammatory diet high in fruits, vegetables, and omega-3 fatty acids, may help to alleviate allergy symptoms. Certain foods, particularly those strong in antioxidants, offer anti-allergic characteristics that may help the body's natural defenses. Individual reactions to dietary changes vary, so it is best to speak with a healthcare practitioner or dietitian before making large changes.

Physical exercise is another important component of overall allergy care. Regular exercise may boost the immune system, lower inflammation, and improve general health. Participating in exercises like yoga or tai chi not only delivers physical advantages, but they also include mindfulness and stress-reduction components, which help with allergy control.

Practical Tips for Everyday Allergy Management.

Allergy-Proofing Your Living Spaces

Creating an allergy-friendly living environment is critical for controlling symptoms and avoiding allergic responses. Simple changes to your living environment may drastically minimize allergy exposure. Consider the following practical methods to allergy-proof your home:

1. Regular cleaning: Common indoor allergies include dust, pet dander, and mold. Regular cleaning, such as dusting surfaces, vacuuming carpets, and cleaning

air filters, may help reduce the occurrence of these allergens.

2. Use allergen-proof bedding. Encase mattresses, pillows, and bedding with allergen-proof coverings to protect against dust mites and other allergens.

3. Control Humidity: Maintain ideal humidity levels (30-50%) to avoid mold formation. Use dehumidifiers in moist locations such as basements and bathrooms.

4. Choose Allergy-Friendly Flooring: Avoid carpets since they may trap allergens. Instead, choose hardwood or tile flooring. If carpets are inevitable, look for

low-pile types and clean them regularly.

5. Limit Indoor Plants: Although plants improve indoor air quality, mold may develop in their soil. Choose plants with little mold spore production or place them in well-ventilated spaces.

CHAPTER SIX
Travel With Allergies: Tips And Tricks

Traveling may provide unique problems for those with allergies, particularly when confronted with strange settings and possible allergens. Whether it's a business trip or a vacation, these tips and methods can make it easier to travel with allergies:

1. Research your destination's allergies before traveling. Knowing the probable triggers helps you to plan and prepare properly.

2. Pack allergy meds: Make sure you have plenty of your recommended medications. Carry them in your carry-on luggage for convenient access throughout the trip.

3. Bring allergy-friendly snacks. Pack allergy-friendly snacks to avoid depending on unfamiliar food choices when traveling. This is especially crucial for those who have food allergies.

4. Notify Accommodations. If you are staying at a hotel or a rental property, notify them of your allergies ahead of time. Many lodgings may provide allergy-

friendly alternatives or make modifications to match your requirements.

5. Carry Allergy Cards: Individuals with severe food allergies may express dietary limitations to restaurant workers using allergy cards in the local language.

Navigating Social Situations With Allergies

Individuals with allergies may find it difficult to interact in social settings, particularly when food is involved. Navigating social gatherings demands efficient communication and proactive techniques to guarantee a safe and pleasurable experience.

1. Communicate allergies clearly: When attending social gatherings, explicitly express your sensitivities to the hosts and other participants. Provide information about particular allergies and cross-contamination dangers.

2. BYO (Bring Your Own): If allergy-friendly alternatives are limited, consider bringing your own to guarantee safe choices.

3. Select Restaurants Wisely When eating out, choose places with allergy-friendly menus or those recognized for accommodating

particular dietary requirements. Call beforehand and discuss your sensitivities with the staff.

4. Be prepared for questions. Prepare to answer inquiries about your allergies and inform people about the seriousness of your illness. This proactive approach may promote understanding and collaboration.

5. Establish an emergency plan: If you have a severe allergic response, always carry your prescription epinephrine auto-injector. Ensure that friends or companions understand how to utilize it in an emergency.

Conclusion

Finally, allergy management goes beyond traditional medical therapies and includes holistic techniques that target both the mind and the body. Mind-body approaches such as meditation and stress management are important in mitigating the effects of allergies because they promote awareness and reduce stress, which may increase symptoms.

Alternative treatments, such as acupuncture and herbal therapy, provide alternative possibilities for those looking for supplementary methods to traditional care. While these treatments should be used under expert supervision, they illustrate the many options for allergy management.

Integrating holistic approaches into traditional therapy stresses the relevance of lifestyle variables in allergy control. Dietary changes, frequent exercise, and stress-reduction tactics improve general well-being and may alleviate allergy symptoms.

Practical suggestions for daily allergy management, such as allergy-proofing living areas, traveling with allergies, and handling social settings, empower people to take control of their allergic symptoms. Individuals who incorporate these tactics into their every day lives may improve their quality of life while reducing the effect of allergies on their overall well-being.